Pressure Cooker Cookbook for Women Over 40

Easy Healthy Dinner Recipes

Patricia J. Powell

Sommario

Introduction

The Ninja Foodi multi-cooker is just one of the devices that every person ought to have in their kitchen area. The device can replace four little tools: slow stove, air fryer, pressure cooker as well as dehydrator.

This recipe book contains several of the dishes we have attempted with the multi-cooker. The dishes range from breakfast, side recipes, chicken, pork, soups, seafood, desserts, and pasta. Additionally, we've put together dozens of vegan recipes you should attempt. We created these dishes taking into consideration newbies and that's why the food preparation treatment is methodical. Besides, the dishes are tasty, delight in reading.

Tomato Basil Soup

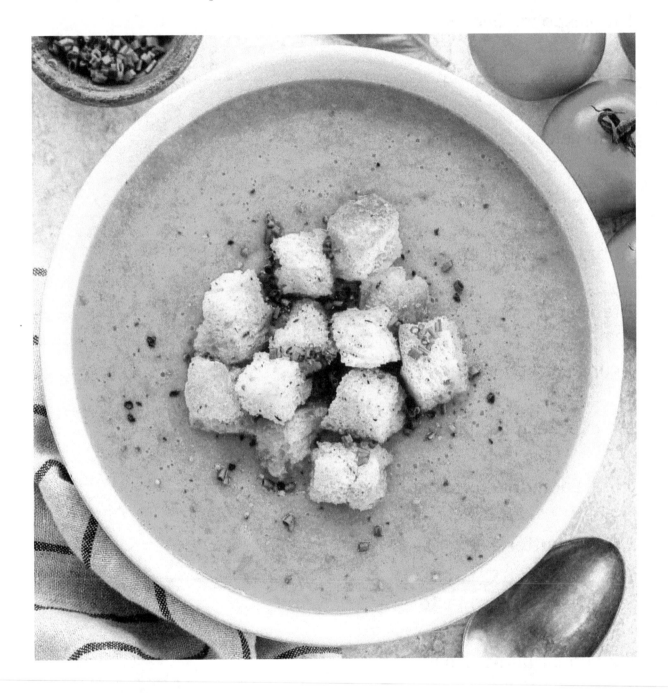

INGREDIENTS (8 Servings)

1 tablespoon olive oil

1 cup onion, chopped

1 cup celery, chopped

1 cup carrot, chopped

30 oz. canned diced tomatoes, undrained

2 tablespoons tomato paste

4 cups chicken broth

1/4 cup fresh basil leaves, chopped

1 teaspoon dried oregano leaves

1/2 cup butter

Salt and pepper to taste

1/2 cup all-purpose flour

1 cup Parmesan cheese, grated

1 1/2 cups half and half

DIRECTIONS (PREP + COOK TIME: 30 MINUTES)

Set the Ninja Foodi to sauté.Pour in the oil.Add the onion, celery and carrot. Cook for 2 minutes. Add the rest of the ingredients except the flour, Parmesan and half and half. Seal the pot. Set it to pressure. Cook at high pressure for 5 minutes.Release the pressure naturally. Pour the soup into a food processor. Pulse until smooth. Pour it back to the pot. Set it to sauté. Add the remaining ingredients.Simmer for 5 minutes. Serving

Kale Chicken Soup

INGREDIENTS (4 Servings)

12 ounces of frozen kale

4 cups of chicken broth

2 glasses of cooked chicken

1 onion, chopped

2 teaspoons of garlic, minced

1 tablespoon of bouillon chicken mix

½ teaspoon of ground cinnamon

1/16 teaspoon of ground cloves

1 teaspoon of salt

1 teaspoon of pepper

DIRECTIONS (PREP + COOK TIME: 20 MINUTES)

Combine all the ingredients in your Foodi and cook on high mode for 5 minutes. Let the pressure escape naturally for 10 minutes and quick release the rest. You can add more seasonings to your chicken soup if necessary.

North African Lentil and Spinach Soup

INGREDIENTS (4-6 Servings)

1 tablespoon of organic olive oil

2 tablespoons of unsalted butter

1 medium red onion, finely chopped

2 teaspoons of ground coriander

1 teaspoon of garlic powder

½ teaspoon of cinnamon powder

¼ teaspoon of clove powder

½ teaspoon of turmeric powder

¼ teaspoon of red pepper cayenne

¼ teaspoon of fresh grated nutmeg

¼ teaspoon of cardamom powder

2 cups of lentils

8 cups of water

¼ teaspoon of pepper

2 teaspoons of salt

6 oz of fresh spinach (about 4 packed cups)

4 tablespoons of freshly squeezed lemon juice

DIRECTIONS (PREP + COOK TIME: 25 MINUTES) Sauté the red onion, ground coriander, garlic powder, cinnamon powder, clove powder, turmeric powder, cayenne pepper, grated nutmeg, and cardamom powder in the melted butter and oil for 2-3 minutes. Add the water and lentils. Close the pressure lid and cook on high mode for 10 minutes. Let the in-built vapor exit naturally and open the lid. Add salt, pepper, and the spinach leaves. Stir to wilt and t add the fresh lemon juice.

Ground Beef Cabbage Soup

INGREDIENTS (14 Servings)A tablespoon of avocado oil

1 large onion, chopped

1 lb of ground beef

A teaspoon of sea salt

1/4 teaspoon of black pepper

1 lb of coleslaw mix, shredded

1 (15-oz) can of diced tomatoes (liquid inclusive)

6 cups of beef bone broth

1 tablespoon of Italian seasoning

1/2 teaspoon of garlic powder

2 medium bay leaves (optional)

DIRECTIONS (PREP + COOK TIME: 45 MINUTES) Sauté the chopped onions in oil for two minutes or until the onions turn translucent while stirring occasionally. Add the ground beef into the Foodi. Add salt and pepper. Sauté on high temperature for 10 minutes while breaking the beef. Add the remaining ingredients and stir. Season the beef with salt and pepper. Close the pressure lid and cook on high mode for 20 minutes Let the pressure release naturally for ten minutes and quick release the rest. Remove the bay leaves and serve.

Chicken Taco Soup Bursting

INGREDIENTS (4 Servings)1 lb of chicken breasts

1/2 cup of onion, diced

A tablespoon of chipotles in adobo sauce, minced

4 garlic cloves, minced

½ teaspoon of chili powder

1 tablespoon of cumin

½ teaspoon of salt

½ teaspoon of paprika

1 tablespoon of lime juice

2 tablespoons of freshly squeezed lemon juice

2 cups of chicken broth

8 ounces of cream cheese

½ cup cilantro, chopped

DIRECTIONS (PREP + COOK TIME: 35 MINUTES) Mix all the ingredients (except the cream cheese and cilantro) in the Foodi. Secure the pressure lid and cook on high mode for 18 minutes. Allow the pressure to exit naturally release for ten minutes and quick release the rest. Remove the chicken with tongs and shred. Set your Foodi to sauté mode and add the cream cheese. Whisk and cook until the cheese dissolves. Turn off the cook function and return the shredded chicken into the pot. Add the cilantro and stir. Serve while topped with cilantro, grated cheddar cheese, diced tomatoes, and sour cream.

Broccoli Cream Soup

INGREDIENTS (4 Servings)

1 head broccoli, cut into florets

4 cups vegetable broth

2 ½ pounds potatoes, peeled and chopped

½ cup heavy cream

⅓ cup butter, melted

1 onion, chopped

2 cloves garlic, minced

½ cup chopped scallions

Ground black pepper and salt to taste

Cheddar cheese to serve

DIRECTIONS (Prep + Cook Time: 15-20 minutes)

Take Ninja Foodi multi-cooker, arrange it over a cooking platform, and open the top lid. In the pot, add the butter; Select "SEAR/SAUTÉ" mode and select "MD: HI" pressure level. Press "STOP/START." After about 4-5 minutes, the butter will start simmering. Add the onions, garlic, and cook (while stirring) for 3-4 minutes until they become softened and translucent. Add the broth, potatoes, and broccoli and mix well. Seal the multi-cooker by locking it with the pressure lid; ensure to keep the pressure release valve locked/sealed. Select "PRESSURE" mode and select the "HI" pressure level. Then, set timer to 5 minutes and press "STOP/START"; it will start the cooking process by building up inside pressure. When the timer goes off, quick release pressure by adjusting the pressure valve to the VENT. After pressure gets released, open the pressure lid. Add the potato mixture in a blender and blend well to puree the mixture. Add the heavy cream and season with pepper and salt to taste; combine well. Serve with scallions and cheese on top.

Double Bean and Ham Soup

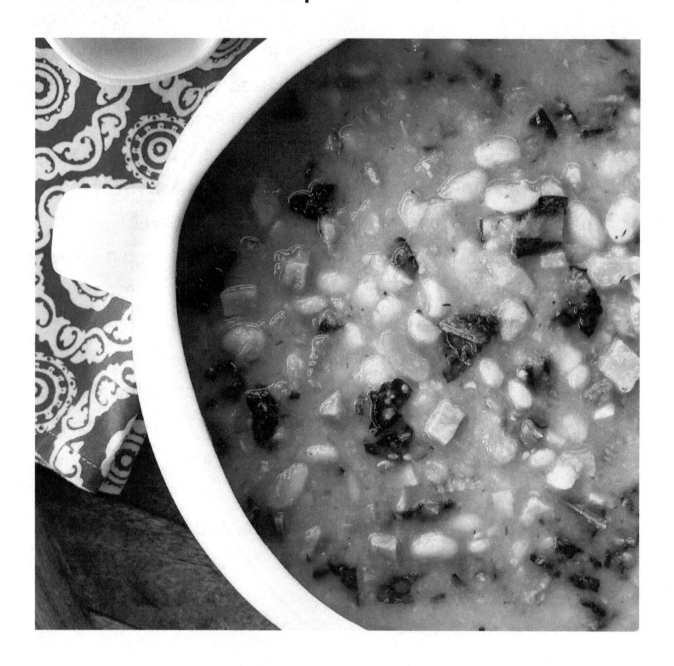

INGREDIENTS (6 Servings)

2 cups of dry navy beans

2 cups of chicken broth

2 cups of water

1 can (14.5 ounce) of diced tomatoes, un-drained

2 carrots, chopped

1 onion, chopped

2 celery stalks, chopped

1 can (16 ounce) of pork and beans, un-drained

A cup of chopped ham

Salt and ground black pepper

DIRECTIONS (PREP + COOK TIME: 55 MINUTES)

Put the chicken broth, navy beans, water carrots, tomatoes, celery, and onion in the Foodi. Close the pressure lid and cook on high mode for 45 minutes. Allow the in-built pressure to exit naturally for 10 minutes and quick release the rest. Open the lid. Add ham, pork, and beans. Stir and season with salt.

Barley and Mushroom Soup

INGREDIENTS (6 Servings)

2 tablespoons of butter

2 carrots (peeled and diced)

1 yellow onion, chopped

3 celery stalks, chopped

2 garlic cloves, minced

1/2 cup of dried mushroom

8 ounces of fresh mushrooms, sliced

6 cups of chicken broth

1/2 cup of pearl barley

2 bay leaves

Salt and pepper

DIRECTIONS (PREP + COOK TIME:420 MINUTES)

Sear your Foodi on medium high heat for a minute. Add butter and melt it. Add carrots and celery and sauté for 2 minutes. Add onion and garlic. Sauté the spice mix for 3 minutes and add the sliced mushrooms. Sauté again for 5 minutes and add the vegetable broth. Stir. Add the barley and bay leaves. Close the pressure lid and cook the ingredients on high mode for 20 minutes. Let the pressure exit naturally and open the lid. Remove the bay leaves and discard. Season your mushroom soup with salt and pepper.

Leek, Potato, and Pea Soup

INGREDIENTS (4 Servings)

2 tablespoons of vegetable oil

1 pound of leeks (washed and chopped finely)

A pound of potatoes, cubed

1 cup of peas

A pinch of dried mint leaves, crumbled

2 tablespoons of fresh parsley, minced

1 cup of coconut milk

4 cups of vegetable stock

Salt and pepper

DIRECTIONS (PREP + COOK TIME: 37 MINUTES)

Sauté the leeks in vegetable oil for ten minutes or until they tender. Add the potatoes, peas, parsley, and mint. Add the coconut milk and the vegetable stock. Add salt and pepper. Close the pressure lid and cook the mixture on high mode for 12 minutes. Quick release the in-built pressure and transfer everything to a mixer. Puree the ingredients and pour your pea soup into bowls.

Beef and Wheat Berry Soup

INGREDIENTS (6 Servings)

2 tablespoon of canola oil

1 onion, chopped finely

A can (6-oz) of tomato paste

4 cups of broth, beef or chicken

1 lb of beef stew or leftover roast, cubed

1/2 cup of wheat berries or barley/brown rice

1 1/2 teaspoon of coarse salt

2 cups of spinach or kale, finely chopped

DIRECTIONS (PREP + COOK TIME: 40 MINUTES) Set your Foodi to sauté mode. Add oil and brown the onions for ten minutes. Add tomato paste and cook-stir for 3 minutes. Add broth, wheat berries, and salt. Cook on high mode for 30 minutes. Quick release the in-built pressure and open the lid. Add the chopped greens and stir.

Butternut Squash and Apple Soup

INGREDIENTS (8 Servings)

1 tablespoon of extra-virgin essential olive oil

3 shallots (peeled and quartered)

1 teaspoon of kosher salt

2 butternut squash-4 lb (peeled, cut, and seeds removed)

2 apples (peeled, cored, and chopped)

1 cup of heavy cream

4 cups of vegetable broth, divided

2 tablespoons of maple syrup

2 teaspoons of apple cider vinegar

Ground black pepper

DIRECTIONS (PREP + COOK TIME: 30 MINUTES) Sauté the shallots in oil for 3 minutes. Add salt and cook until it turns brown. Add apples, butternut squash, and a cup of broth. Stir. Close the pressure lid and cook on high mode for 5 minutes. Quick release the in-built pressure and open the lid. Add cream and the reserved broth. Puree the ingredients using an immersion blender. Add maple syrup and vinegar. Sauté on low mode until the soup is well-heated. Add salt and pepper.

Chinese Hot and Sour Soup

INGREDIENTS (8 Servings)

DIRECTIONS (PREP + COOK TIME: 20 MINUTES)

1 lb of pork tenderloin, sliced thinly

1 lb of extra firm tofu

5 cups of chicken broth

1 cup of dried mushrooms

4 eggs, lightly beaten

3 tablespoons of soy sauce

3 tablespoons of water

2 tablespoons of Chinese rice vinegar or white vinegar

1 tablespoon of Chinese black vinegar

1 teaspoon of salt

2 teaspoons of ground pepper

½ teaspoon of xantham gum

DIRECTIONS (PREP + COOK TIME: 20 MINUTES)

Mix all the ingredients (except tofu and eggs) in the pot. Close the pressure lid and cook on high mode for ten minutes. Let the pressure release naturally for 10 minutes and quick release the rest. Reset the Foodi to sauté mode and remove the mushroom. Slice it thinly and return it to the Foodi. Add the tofu and stir. Add the eggs gently and stir thrice, preferably with chopsticks. Close the pressure lid and cook for a minute. Serve. Belize

Keto No- Beans Chili

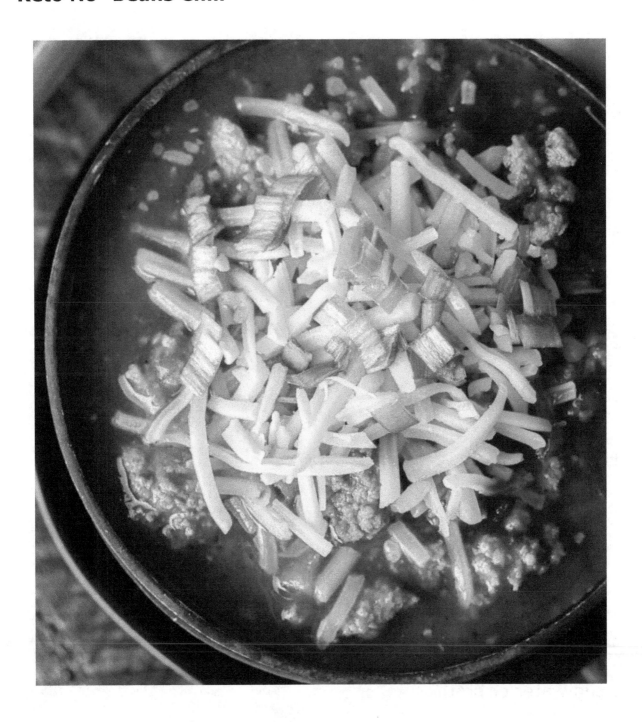

INGREDIENTS (10 Servings)

2 1/2 lbs of ground beef

1/2 large onion, chopped

8 garlic cloves, minced

2 cans (15-oz) of diced tomatoes (liquid inclusive)

1 can (6-oz) of tomato paste

1 can (4-oz) of green chilies (liquid inclusive)

2 tablespoons of Worcestershire sauce

2 tablespoons of cumin

1/4 cup of chili powder

1 tablespoons of dried oregano

1 teaspoon of black pepper

2 teaspoons of sea salt

1 cup water or broth

DIRECTIONS (PREP + COOK TIME: 65 MINUTES)

Set your Ninja Foodi to sauté mode. Add a little oil and the chopped onion and cook until they become translucent. Add the garlic and cook until fragrant. Add the ground beef and cook-stir until they turn brown. Add the remaining ingredients (except bay leaf) and close the pressure lid. Cook on high mode for 30 minutes. When the cooking duration elapses, let the in-built steam escape naturally and open the lid.

Vegetable Soup

INGREDIENTS (6 Servings)

1 tablespoon of extra-virgin organic olive oil

4 garlic cloves, minced

1 medium onion, chopped

Kosher salt   Freshly ground black pepper

1 tablespoon of tomato paste

2 cups of chopped cabbage

2 cups of small cauliflower florets

2 celery stalks, thinly sliced

2 carrots (peeled and thinly sliced)

1 red bell pepper, chopped

1 medium zucchini, chopped

A can (15-oz) of kidney beans (rinsed and drained)

1 can (15-oz) of diced tomatoes

4 cups of vegetable broth, low-sodium

3/4 teaspoon of paprika

2 teaspoons of Italian seasoning

Freshly parsley, chopped for serving

DIRECTIONS (PREP + COOK TIME:55 MINUTES)

Sauté the chopped onion and garlic in oil. Add some salt and pepper. Cook-stir for 5 minutes or until the onion softens. Add tomato paste and cook for a minute while stirring. Add the remaining ingredients and stir to mix. Close the pressure lid and cook for 12 minutes. Quick release the in-built pressure and open the lid. Season with salt and pepper. Add parsley and essential olive oil.

Carrot Ginger and Turmeric Soup

INGREDIENTS (6 Servings)

A teaspoon of canola oil

1 large yellow onion, diced

3 garlic cloves, minced

1 ginger piece, (about an inch,) peeled and chopped

2 celery stalks, chopped

3 cups of carrots (peeled and chopped)

1/4 teaspoon of ground turmeric

3 cups of chicken stock

1 teaspoon of sea salt

1/3 cup of heavy cream

2 tablespoon of chopped cilantro

Freshly ground pepper, for serving

DIRECTIONS (PREP + COOK TIME: 15 MINUTES)

Set your Ninja Foodi to sauté mode and heat it for 5 minutes. Add oil and brown the onions. Add the garlic and cook for a minute. Add the carrots, ginger, celery, and turmeric. Stir. Close the pressure lid and cook on high mode for 6 minutes. Quick release the in-built pressure and open the lid. Puree the soup ingredients and add cream and black pepper. Blend again. Serve with cream and cilantro.

Zucchini Pasta Sauce

INGREDIENTS (5 Servings)

3 medium zucchinis, chopped

1 tablespoon of olive oil

2 garlic cloves, minced finely

Pinch of crushed red pepper

3/4 cup of water

1/4 cup of fresh basil leaves

2 tablespoons of pine nuts

Salt and black pepper

16 oz of pasta, cooked

1 tablespoon of vegetable essential olive oil

DIRECTIONS (PREP + COOK TIME: 13 MINUTES)

Preheat your Foodi by sautéing it on medium high for 5 minutes. Heat the oil and add garlic and the crushed red pepper. Sauté for 2 minutes and add the zucchini. Pour water into the Foodi and add salt and pepper. Close the pressure lid and cook on high mode for 3 minutes. Quick release the in-built pressure and open the lid. Add the pine nuts and basil leaves. Stir. Transfer everything into a blender and puree. Serve your zucchini pasta sauce with cooked pasta swirled with vegetable oil.

Chicken and Vegetable Noodle Soup

INGREDIENTS (4 Servings)

2 tablespoons of coconut oil

1 pound of boneless and skinless chicken thighs

1 cup of diced carrots

1 cup of diced celery

¾ cup of green onions, chopped

6 cups of chicken stock

½ teaspoon of dried oregano

½ teaspoon of dried basil

1/8 teaspoon of fresh ground pepper

1 teaspoon of grey sea salt

2 cups of spiralized daikon noodles

DIRECTIONS (PREP + COOK TIME: 30 MINUTES)

Preheat your Ninja Foodi on sauté mode for two minutes. Add some coconut oil into the pot and brown the chicken thighs. Shred the chicken using a fork and then add the carrots, celery, and onions. Let it cook for two minutes and add the remaining ingredients. Close the pressure lid and cook on high mode for 15 minutes. Quick release the in-built pressure and open the lid. Add the add daikon noodles and serve.

Homemade Hot Sauce

INGREDIENTS (2 Servings)

12 oz of fresh hot peppers, chopped

1 medium onion, minced

3 garlic cloves, minced

A teaspoon of extra virgin olive oil

1 teaspoon of kosher salt

A cup of apple cider vinegar

1/2 cup of water

DIRECTIONS (PREP + COOK TIME: 15 MINUTES)

Sauté the garlic, onion, vinegar, and salt for three minutes in your Foodi pot. Add water and close the pressure lid. Cook for on high mode for one minute and let the pressure exit naturally. Transfer the mixture into an immersion blender and Puree. Add more seasonings if necessary and puree again. Pour the mixture into a glass jar and let it rest for 3 days before using. You can refrigerate your hot sauce for months.

Chili Queso Chicken Soup

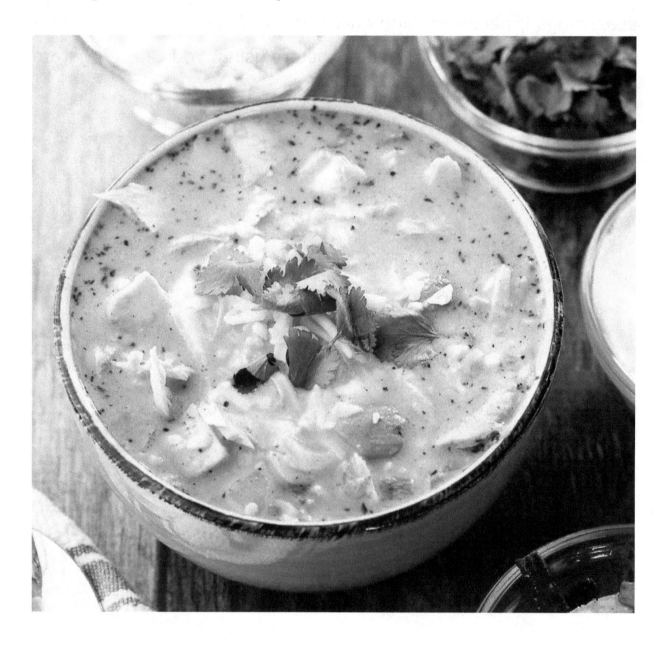

INGREDIENTS (6 Servings)

2 chicken breast pieces (boneless and skinless)

28 oz of diced tomatoes

1/4 teaspoon of salt

1 cup of green salsa

2 cups of chicken broth

2 tablespoons of taco seasoning

8 ounces of softened cream cheese

DIRECTIONS (PREP + COOK TIME:35 MINUTES) Mix the chicken with juicy tomatoes, green salsa, taco seasoning, chicken broth, and salt in the Foodi. Close the pressure lid and cook for10 minutes. Let the pressure escape naturally for 15 minutes. Remove the chicken pieces and transfer them on a platter. Add the creamy cheese and stir until it's heated. Add the chicken pieces and serve with avocado and cheese.

Tortellini Soup

INGREDIENTS (4 Servings)

A tablespoon of garlic, minced

1 tablespoon of dried onion, minced

A tablespoon of chicken base

½ teaspoon of pepper, coarsely ground

1 ½ pounds of fresh carrots (peeled and cut into ¼ inch coins)

6 ounces of dried cheese tortellini

¼ cup of dry white wine

6 cups of chicken stock

7 oz of fresh baby spinach (cleaned and stem removed)

Parmesan cheese for garnishing

DIRECTIONS (PREP + COOK TIME: 22 MINUTES) Combine the onions with garlic, chicken base, and ground pepper in your Foodi pot. Add the carrots and spread the tortellini on top. Pour the chicken broth and white wine in the Pot. Close the pressure lid and cook on high mode for two minutes. Quick release the in-built steam and open the Foodi. Add the spinach and stir. Allow it to rest for two minutes. Enjoy your soup with the parmesan cheese.

Creamy Tomato Feta Soup

INGREDIENTS (6 Servings)

2 tablespoons of organic olive oil or butter

1/4 cup of onion, chopped

2 garlic cloves

1/8 teaspoon of black pepper

1/2 teaspoon of salt

A teaspoon of pesto sauce, optional

1/2 teaspoon of dried oregano

A teaspoon of dried basil

1 tablespoon of tomato paste, optional

10 tomatoes (skinned, seeded, and chopped)

3 glasses of water

1/3 cup of almond milk

2/3 cup of feta cheese, crumbled

DIRECTIONS (PREP + COOK TIME: 20 MINUTES) Preheat your Foodi by sautéing it over medium high heat for 5 minutes. Heat the olive oil and add the onion. Stir and cook for a minute. Add the garlic and cook for another minute. Add the tomatoes, pepper, salt, optional pesto, oregano, tomato paste, basil, and water. Close the pressure lid and cook on high mode for 15 minutes. Let the pressure exit naturally and open the lid. Pour everything into an immersion blender and puree. Add the feta cheese and almond milk and simmer on low mode for three minutes minute. Serve your feta soup warm.

Spicy Pasta Sauce

INGREDIENTS (4 Servings)

3 tablespoons of canola oil

1 medium onion, chopped

4 garlic cloves, chopped

1 can (28-oz) of crushed tomatoes

A tablespoon of dried dill

2 tablespoons of dried basil

1 tablespoon of dried thyme

1/4 teaspoon of crushed red pepper flakes

2 teaspoons of dried oregano

1/3 cup of dry dark wine

1/2 cup of water 1 bay leaf

DIRECTIONS (PREP + COOK TIME: 25 MINUTES)

Preheat your Ninja Foodi on sauté mode over medium high for 5 minutes. Sauté the onions and garlic. Add the remaining ingredients and stir. Close the pressure lid and cook for 10 minutes. Quick release the in-built pressure and open the lid. Serve the spicy pasta with cooked pasta.

Beans Chicken Chili

INGREDIENTS (4 Servings)

2 cans (15-oz) of great Northern beans, drained

4 cups of cooked and shredded chicken

2 cups of Salsa Verde

6 glasses of chicken stock

2 teaspoons of ground cumin

DIRECTIONS (PREP + COOK TIME: 13 MINUTES)

Add all the ingredients (except the beans) in the pot. Close the pressure lid and cook the mixture on high mode for 8 minutes. Quick release the in-built vapor and open the lid. Add beans and stir.

Chicken Thigh Soup

. INGREDIENTS (6 Servings)

 4 celery stalks, chopped

10 oz of radishes

1/2 small onion, chopped

1 tablespoon of fresh basil, chopped

A tablespoon of fresh rosemary, chopped

3 cloves of garlic, minced

1/2 teaspoon of salt

1/4 teaspoon of ground black pepper

4 glasses of chicken broth

2 pounds of chicken thighs (skin and bones on)

2 bay leaves

Fresh parsley for garnish

DIRECTIONS (PREP + COOK TIME: 40 MINUTES) Add the chopped celery stalks, rosemary, radishes, garlic, basil, onion, salt, and pepper in your Foodi pot. Pour the chicken broth over the vegetables and stir. Add the chicken thighs and bay leaves. Close the pressure lid and cook on high mode for 30 minutes. Allow the in-built steam to escape naturally for 15 minutes and quick release the rest. Remove the chicken using tongs and separate fresh parts from the bones and skins. Subdivide it into pieces and return them to the Foodi. Add more seasonings if necessary. Subdivide your chicken thigh soup into bowls and serve. Top with fresh parsley and enjoy.

White Chicken Chili

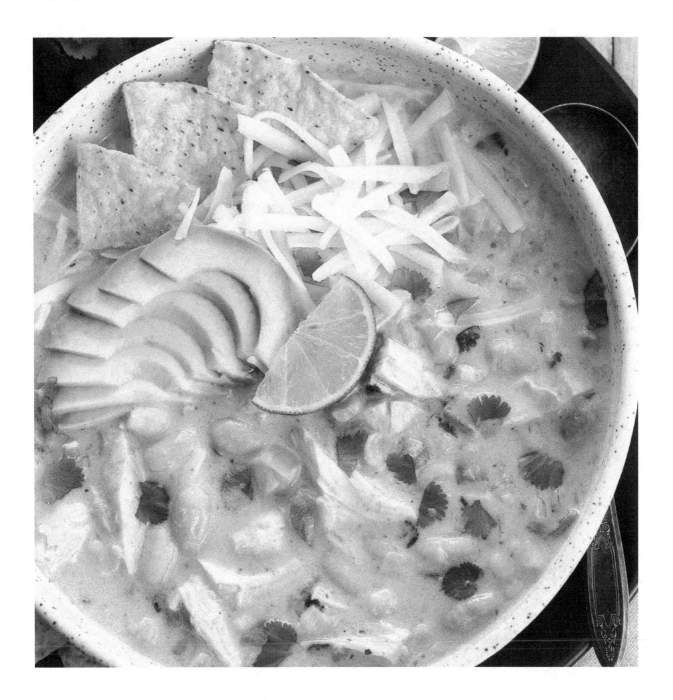

INGREDIENTS (4 Servings)

11/2 lbs of chicken white meat

2 garlic cloves

1 cup of celery, chopped

A cup of onion, chopped

1 cup of heavy cream

1 tablespoon of Poblano pepper

3 glasses of chicken broth

1 cup of water

A tablespoon of cumin

1 tablespoon of turmeric

Salt and pepper

Coconut or avocado oil

DIRECTIONS (PREP + COOK TIME: 30 MINUTES) Pour water
into the Foodi pot. Put the chicken in the basket and fix it into the

pot. Close the pressure lid and cook it on high pressure for 12 minutes. Allow the pressure to escape naturally and open the lid. Remove the chicken using tongs and shred it into pieces. Sauté the avocado oil in your Foodi on medium high heat for one minute. Add the diced onions, poblano pepper, garlic, and celery. Sauté them until the onion turns light brown. Add broth and water to the mixture. Allow it to simmer and add the chicken spices followed by heavy cream. Mix them well. Close the pressure lid and cook the mixture on high mode for 3 minutes. Quick release the in-built pressure and serve.

Kimchi Beef Stew

INGREDIENTS (6 Servings)

1 pound of beef cubes, cut

2 glasses of kimchi

2 cups of water

1 cup of chopped firm tofu, optional

1 cup of dried shiitake mushrooms

1 cup of chopped onion

½ cup of chopped green onion(optional)

1 tablespoon of dark soy sauce

A tablespoon of crushed ginger

1 tablespoon of crushed garlic

1 tablespoon of Gochujang

A tablespoon of sesame oil

1 tablespoon of Gochugaru Korean chili paste

½ teaspoon of sugar   Salt

DIRECTIONS (PREP + COOK TIME: 25 MINUTES) Mix all the ingredients in the Foodi and cook on high mode for 15 minutes. Let the pressure release naturally for 5 minutes. Add the tofu and green onions. Serve hot. Oxtails Stew Preparation time: 10minutes| Cook Time: 15| Servings: 4 Ingredients 5 pounds of oxtails 2 glasses of red 1 large onion (peeled and chopped) 3 carrots, chopped 3 celery stalks, chopped 1 cup of chopped tomatoes 1 small parsley, chopped A garlic clove (peeled and chopped) 1 cup of water Sugar Salt and pepper Directions Begin by seasoning the oxtails with salt and pepper. Put them into the Ninja Foodi. Add the remaining ingredients (except wine and water) into the oxtails. Add the wine and water. Cook the ingredients on high mode for 10 minutes. Allow the pressure to escape naturally and open the lid. Add more seasonings, if required. Enjoy!

Minestrone Soup

INGREDIENTS (6 Servings)

2 tablespoons of canola oil

4 cloves garlic (peeled and sliced thinly)

2 celery stalks, chopped

1 medium yellow onion (peeled and chopped)

Pinch red pepper, crushed

1 teaspoon of ground black pepper

2 teaspoons of kosher salt

2 medium carrots (peeled and chopped)

2 Yukon Gold potatoes (peeled and diced)

1/2 teaspoon of dried thyme

1 can (14.5 oz) of diced tomatoes

1/2 teaspoon of dried oregano

2 bay leaves 4 cups of broth (chicken or vegetable)

2 cups of water

1 can (15 oz.) of red kidney beans (rinsed and drained)

2 cups of baby spinach

2 teaspoons of lemon juice

Fresh Parmesan cheese, grated

DIRECTIONS (PREP + COOK TIME: 21 MINUTES) Preheat the Ninja unit for 5 minutes. Sauté oil, garlic, celery, crushed red pepper, pepper, and salt. Stir and cook until everything softens. Add the remaining ingredients (except Parmesan) and cook for a minute on high mode. Quick release the in-built pressure and open the lid. Serve while topped with Parmesan Cheese.

Potato Leek Soup

INGREDIENTS (6 Servings)

2 tablespoon of butter

2 leeks (white and green,) sliced

1/2 teaspoon of kosher salt

3 garlic cloves, minced

1/2 teaspoon of dried thyme

1 bay leaf 1 1/2 lb of yellow potatoes (peeled and diced)

5 cups of low sodium stock (vegetable or chicken)

1 cup of half and half

Kosher salt and black pepper

Optional toppings:

chives croutons cream bacon

DIRECTIONS (PREP + COOK TIME: 55 MINUTES) Set your Ninja Foodi to sauté mode. Let it preheat for two minutes. Add butter and melt. Add the leeks and sauté it for 8 minutes. Add the garlic and cook for a minute. Add the potatoes, thyme, bay leaf, and stock. Close the pressure lid and cook on high mode for 7 minutes Let the pressure release naturally for 10 minutes and quick release the rest. Open the lid and remove the bay leaf. Puree everything using a blender. Add the half and half and more seasonings if required. Serve your soup with the optional toppings.

Chicken and Kale Stew Tender.

INGREDIENTS (4 Servings)

1 tablespoon of butter

½ of a medium chopped onion

2 boneless chicken breasts, diced

3 cups of kale, chopped

1 can (14.5 oz.) of diced tomatoes

A cup of chicken broth

1/2 teaspoon of garlic powder

1/2 teaspoon of salt

1/2 teaspoon of oregano

1/4 teaspoon of ground black pepper

DIRECTIONS (PREP + COOK TIME: 40 MINUTES) Set your Foodi to sauté mode. Add butter and melt. Add the onion and cook for 3 minutes or until tender. Now, add the chicken and cook until crispy. Add the chicken broth, kale, diced tomatoes, garlic powder, oregano, salt, and black pepper into the pot contents. Close the pressure lid and cook on high mode for ten minutes. Quick release the in-built pressure and open the lid.

Homemade Marinara Sauce

INGREDIENTS (6 Servings)

4 tablespoons of olive oil

3 garlic cloves, minced

1/3 cup of onions, diced

2 large carrots, diced

3 tablespoons of chopped fresh parsley

1 can (28-oz) of whole tomatoes, crushed

A teaspoon of dried oregano

1/4 teaspoon of ground black pepper

1/2 teaspoon of dried thyme

1/2 teaspoon of salt

DIRECTIONS (PREP + COOK TIME: 45 MINUTES)

Preheat the Foodi unit on sauté mode. Add the onion and garlic in oil. Cook for two minutes and add the carrots. Cook for two minutes and add the crushed tomatoes (juice inclusive,) parsley, thyme, oregano, pepper, and salt. Secure the pressure lid and cook on high mode for 30 minutes. Quick release the in-built pressure and open the lid. Serve.

Pot Roast Soup

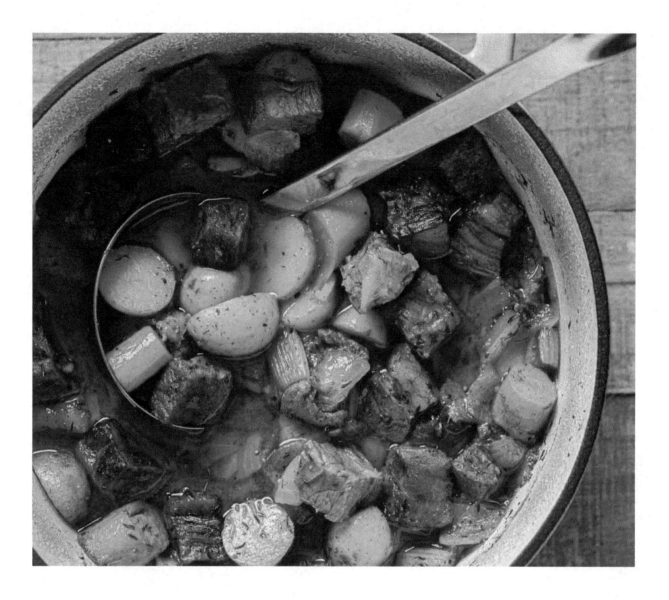

INGREDIENTS (6 Servings)

2 lbs of chuck roast, cubed

½ teaspoon of black pepper

½ teaspoon of kosher salt

2 tablespoons of organic olive oil

3 carrots (peeled and chopped)

1 white onion, chopped

2 celery stalks, chopped

1 green pepper, chopped

4 garlic cloves

1/3 cup of farro

4 glasses of beef stock

¼ cup of tomato paste

Salt and pepper

A teaspoon of dried thyme

DIRECTIONS (PREP + COOK TIME: 50 MINUTES)

Season the cubed roast with salt and pepper. Brown the seasoned roast on sauté mode. Remove and set aside. Add the vegetables and cook for 6-7 minutes. Remove and set aside. Return the browned beef into the Foodi and add the farro, tomato paste, thyme, and beef stock. Close the pressure lid and cook on high mode for twenty minutes. Let the pressure exit naturally for 5 minutes and quick release the rest. Open lid and return the cooked veggies. Simmer on sauté for three minutes and serve hot.

Chicken Stew

INGREDIENTS (8 Servings)

DIRECTIONS (PREP + COOK TIME: 40 MINUTES)

4 whole chicken legs (cut into 8 pieces)

2 glasses of chicken stock

1 cup of yellow onions, sliced

2 tablespoons of white wine vinegar

3 tablespoons of Worcestershire sauce

2 tablespoons of achiote paste

1 tablespoon of coconut oil

1 tablespoon of granulated sugar substitute

3 cloves of garlic, sliced

1 teaspoon of Mexican dried oregano

½ teaspoon of ground black pepper

DIRECTIONS (PREP + COOK TIME: 40 MINUTES)

Combine the achiote with vinegar, cumin, oregano, sweetener, Worcestershire sauce, and pepper in a bowl. Rub the chicken with the achiote mixture and marinate it overnight. Preheat the Foodi pot on sauté mode and brown the chicken in oil. Transfer it to a bowl and reserve the marinade. Sauté the onions and garlic until tender. Return the chicken to the pot. Combine the broth and the reversed marinade and pour into the Foodi. Close the pressure lid and cook on high mode for 20 minutes. Release the in-built pressure and open the lid.

Tomato Basil Soup

INGREDIENTS (8 Servings)

3 tablespoons of olive oil

3 garlic cloves, minced

2 yellow onions, chopped

3 1/2 cups of vegetable broth

3 pounds of tomatoes, quartered

1 tablespoon of tomato paste

2 cups of fresh basil leaves, lightly packed

1 teaspoon of fresh thyme leaves

1/2 teaspoon of freshly ground black pepper

1/2 teaspoon of salt

1/4 cups of grated cheese

DIRECTIONS (PREP + COOK TIME: 45 MINUTES)

Preheat the Foodi unit on Sauté mode. Add the essential olive oil and sauté the onions until they tenderize. Add the garlic and cook for a minute. Add the vegetable broth, tomato paste, tomatoes, thyme, basil, salt, and pepper. Close the pressure lid and cook on high mode for 5 minutes. Quick release the remaining pressure and open the lid. Puree the ingredients using an immersion. Add Parmesan and simmer on sauté mode for 4 minutes.

African Lamb Stew

INGREDIENTS (6 Servings)

2 pounds of boneless lamb shoulder

1 tablespoon of canola oil

1 cup of dried apricots, cut into four

2 cloves of garlic (peeled and minced)

1 large onion (peeled and diced)

1/3 cup of raisins

1 tablespoon of minced fresh ginger

1/3 cup of blanched almonds

½ teaspoon of ground cinnamon

1/3 cup of fresh mint leaves, packed

¾ cup of red wine

¼ cup of fresh orange juice

Fresh mint leaves, optional for garnish

Salt and freshly ground pepper

DIRECTIONS (PREP + COOK TIME: 50 MINUTES)

Preheat the Foodi unit on sauté mode. Trim the lamb of fat and cut it into pieces. Brown the lamb pieces in oil and set aside. Add the onion and sauté for 3 minutes. Add the garlic and sauté for 30 seconds. Add the browned lamb and stir. Add the raisins, apricots, ginger, almonds, wine, cinnamon, mint leaves, and orange juice. Close the pressure lid and cook on high mode for 20 minutes. Quick release the in-built pressure and garnish if desired. Serve your lamb stew alongside couscous.

French Onion Soup

INGREDIENTS (4 Servings)

2 tablespoons of butter

2 large white onions, (peeled and sliced, 1/4-inches)

1 tablespoon of soy sauce

A tablespoon of tomato paste

1 tablespoon of Worcestershire sauce

A box (32 oz) of beef stock

1 teaspoon of ground black pepper

A teaspoon of kosher salt

4 cups of crusty French bread (cubed into 1" pieces)

2 cups of Mozzarella cheese, shredded

DIRECTIONS (PREP + COOK TIME: 60 MINUTES)

Preheat the Foodi unit for 5 minutes on sauté mode. Add onions and butter. Cook-stir the onions for ten minutes. Add the soy sauce, tomato paste, and Worcestershire sauce. Cook for 5 minutes and add stock, pepper, and salt. Close the pressure lid and cook on high mode for 15 minutes. Quick release the in-built pressure and open the lid. Sprinkle the bread cubes over the soup, squeeze the cheese in the bread. Close the crisping lid and broil for 8 minutes.

Chinese Pork Soup

INGREDIENTS (6 Servings)

1 pound of pork shoulder, chunked

3 cups of chopped bok Choy

¼ cup of cilantro

3 cups of water

6 garlic cloves, crushed

3-inch crushed ginger

2 tablespoons of black vinegar

2 tablespoons of peanut oil

2 tablespoons of doban Jiang paste

2 tablespoons of soy sauce

½ onion, sliced

2 teaspoons of Szechuan pepper, coarsely crushed

11/2 teaspoons of sugar

11/2 teaspoons of salt

DIRECTIONS (PREP + COOK TIME: 45 MINUTES)

Sauté the garlic and ginger on your Foodi. Add the onion, vinegar, soy sauce, pork, doban Jiang paste, water, sugar, salt, and pepper. Seal the pressure lid and cook on high mode for 10 minutes. Quick release the in-built steam and open the lid. Add the bok Choy and cover. Let your pork soup sit for ten minutes. Serve while garnished with cilantro.

Zuppa Toscana Soup

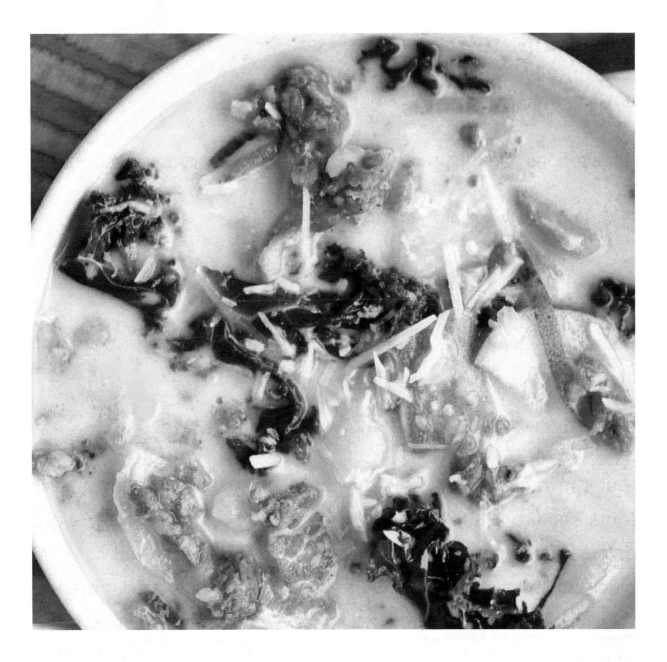

INGREDIENTS (10 Servings)

1 lb of mild Italian sausage

A bag (16 oz) of whole radishes

1 medium onion, diced

2 teaspoons of garlic, minced 32 oz of broth, chicken or vegetable

⅓ Cup of heavy cream

4 cups of kale leaves

DIRECTIONS (PREP + COOK TIME: 45 MINUTES)

Cut the radishes into small chunks. Add the sausage to your Ninja Foodi pot and sauté until browned. Pour the broth, diced onions, garlic, and radishes. Close the pressure lid and cook on high mode for fifteen minutes. Let the accumulated pressure release naturally and open the lid. Add the heavy cream and the torn kale leaves. Sauté the mixture for 3 minutes to soften the kale.

Italian Chicken, Lentil, and Bacon Stew

INGREDIENTS (4 Servings)

2 1/2 pounds of chicken pieces (bone and skin-on)

8 oz of pancetta, cut into 1/2-inch

2 tablespoons of canola oil

2 medium carrots (peeled and chopped)

1 medium onion, diced (about 1 cup)

2 bay leaves 2 teaspoons of sherry vinegar

8 oz of dried French lentils

12 sprigs of parsley

4 cups of chicken stock

Kosher salt and freshly ground black pepper

DIRECTIONS (PREP + COOK TIME: 30 MINUTES)

Chop the leaves and parsley roughly and tie their stems using a twine. Sauté the bacon until crispy and then add the onions. Cook until they soften and add the chicken stock, lentils, carrots, stems, bay leaves, parsley and the chicken legs. Season the legs mix with salt and pepper. Stir. Close the pressure lid and cook on high mode for 20 minutes. Quick release the in-built pressure and open the lid. Transfer your chicken into a bowl and discard the parsley stems. Sauté the lentil mixture until it thickens. Shred the chicken and discard the bones and skin. Add chicken and vinegar to the beans and stir. Season the boneless and skinless chicken pieces with salt and pepper. Add half of the chopped parsley and stir. Serve while topped with olive oil, parsley, and sherry vinegar.

Beef Taco Soup

INGREDIENTS (8 Servings)

2 lbs of ground beef

1 tablespoon of onion flakes, optional

4 garlic cloves, minced

2 tablespoons of chili powder

2 teaspoons of cumin

20 oz of diced tomatoes with chilies (Rotel)

32 oz of beef broth

Salt and pepper

8 oz of creamy cheese

1/2 cup of heavy cream

Optional Toppings:

Sliced black olives

Sour cream Cheddar cheese, shredded

Sliced jalapeño peppers

DIRECTIONS (PREP + COOK TIME: 25 MINUTES)

Set your Foodi to sauté mode. Add the ground beef and brown it for 5 minutes. Add the diced tomatoes with chili, onion flakes, chili powder, garlic, beef broth, cumin, salt, and pepper.   Close the pressure lid and cook on high mode for 5 minutes. Let the pressure escape naturally for 10 minutes and quick release the rest. Open the lid and add the creamy cheese and cheese. You can serve with the optional toppings.

Mexican Pork Soup

INGREDIENTS (S12ervings)

36 oz of shredded pork shoulder

2 cups of cooked pumpkin

6 tablespoons of pork lard

6 cups of chicken broth

1 cup of cilantro, chopped

1 lime, cut

A cup of canned green chili, chopped

4 avocados, diced

2 teaspoons of ground cumin

1 teaspoon of paprika, smoked

2 teaspoons of garlic powder

1 teaspoon of sea salt

1 onion, diced

4 cups of kale, chopped

DIRECTIONS (PREP + COOK TIME: 40 MINUTES)

Mix the cumin with garlic powder, paprika, and salt in a bowl. Preheat the Foodi unit and add the pork lard, onion, pork shoulder, green chili, pumpkin, broth, and the spice mix. Close the pressure lid and cook on high mode for 30 minutes. Let the accumulated vapor exit naturally and open the lid. Add the kale and serve with avocado and cilantro toppings. You can

garnish with lime.

Bacon Cheeseburger Soup

INGREDIENTS (6 Servings)

1 pound of lean ground beef

1/2 can of fire-roasted tomatoes

3 glasses of beef broth

1/4 cup of cooked and crumbled bacon

1 tablespoon of pickled jalapenos, chopped

2 teaspoons of Worcestershire sauce

4 oz of cream cheese

1 cup of sharp cheddar cheese, shredded

1/2 medium onion, diced

1 teaspoon of salt

1/2 teaspoon of pepper

1/2 teaspoon of garlic powder

A pickled spear, diced

DIRECTIONS (PREP + COOK TIME: 20 MINUTES)

Preheat your Ninja Foodi on medium high for two minutes. Sauté the ground beef and onion for 5 minutes. Add the tomatoes, bacon, broth, garlic powder, Worcestershire sauce, the jalapenos, salt, and pepper. Add cream cheese and stir. Close the pressure lid and cook the mixture on high mode for 15 minutes. Quick release the in-built pressure and open the lid. Serve your cheeseburger soup while garnished with diced shredded cheddar and pickles.

Chicken Zoodle Soup

INGREDIENTS (6 Servings)

3 celery stalks, diced

2 tablespoons of pickled jalapeño, diced

1 cup bok Choy, sliced

3 zucchinis, spiralized

½ cup of fresh spinach

1 tablespoon of coconut oil

¼ medium onion, diced

¼ cup of button mushrooms, diced

2 cups of cooked chicken, diced

3 cups of chicken broth

1 bay leaf

½ teaspoon of garlic powder

1 teaspoon of salt

⅛teaspoon of cayenne

DIRECTIONS (PREP + COOK TIME: 25 MINUTES) Preheat your Foodi by sautéing it on medium heat for two minutes. Add coconut oil, onions, and mushrooms. Sauté the mixture for 5 minutes or until it produce a sweet smell. Add the celery, spinach, jalapeños, and bok Choy. Cook for 4 minutes and switch off the sauté mode. Add mushrooms and onion. Sauté for 3 to 4 minutes or until the onion becomes translucent and fragrant. Add celery and spinach. Cook for 4 minutes and open the lid. Add the cooked chicken, broth, seasonings, and bay leaf. Close the pressure lid and cook on high mode for 20 minutes. Release the inbuilt pressure naturally for ten minutes and quick release the rest. Open the lid and add the spiralised zucchini. Sauté the zucchini mixture on low mode for 3 minutes or until they tenderize. Enjoy warm!

Wild Rice Soup

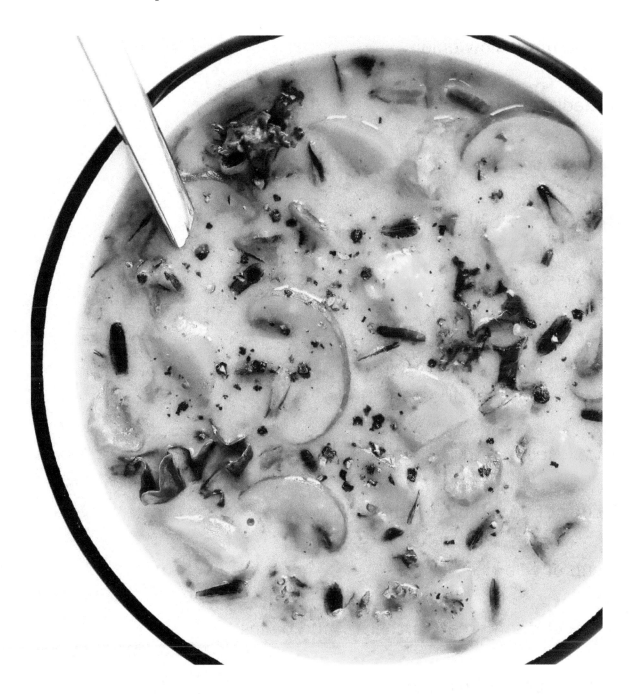

INGREDIENTS (8 Servings)

1/2 cup of raw cashews

1 medium yellow onion

4 medium carrots

2 celery stalks

8 oz of baby Bella mushrooms

6 cloves of garlic

2 tablespoons of extra virgin olive oil

2 tablespoons of dried oregano

1 tablespoon of dried thyme

8 cups of vegetable broth

1 cup of wild rice

A cup of dried great northern white beans

1/2 teaspoon of black pepper

2 1/2 teaspoons of kosher salt, divided

2 teaspoons of dried sage

1 tablespoon of soy sauce, tamari, or liquid aminos

DIRECTIONS (PREP + COOK TIME: 80 MINUTES)

Soak the cashews in water. Dice the onion, slice the celery and mushrooms, cut the carrots roundly, and mince the garlic. Sauté the onion, celery, and carrot in oil for 5 minutes. Add mushrooms and cook for 2 minutes. Add the garlic, oregano, and thyme. Cook and stir for 2 minutes. Add the broth, dried white beans, wild rice, black pepper, and kosher salt. Close the pressure lid and cook on high mode for 50 minutes. Quick release the in-built pressure and transfer 2 cups of the pot's content into a blender. Drain the soaked cashews and add them into the blender. Add the dried sage. Puree and repeat the procedure with the remaining beans mixture. Add the soy sauce and ½ teaspoon of kosher salt. Garnish with the essential olive oil and ground pepper. Enjoy!

Cauliflower Soup

INGREDIENTS (6 Servings)

6 slices of bacon, chopped

3 glasses of chicken broth

1½ glasses of cheese -cheddar or Monterey, shredded

¼ cup of onion, chopped

¾ cup of sour cream

1 green onion

2 garlic cloves, crushed

A cauliflower head, cut into pieces

1 celery stalk, chopped

Salt and Pepper

DIRECTIONS (PREP + COOK TIME: 40 MINUTES)

Sauté the bacon slices while stirring frequently and transfer them to a paper- lined plate, once crispy.   Add the onion, garlic, celery, salt, and pepper. Cook until they soften and turn off the sauté mode.   Add broth and the cauliflower florets. Close the pressure lid and cook on high mode for 5 minutes. Let the accumulated steam escape naturally for ten minutes and quick release the rest. Add a cup of cheese and cream. Pour everything into an immersion blender and puree. Add the bacon, green onion, and cheese for the topping.

Spicy Cranberry Sauce

INGREDIENTS (21/4 Servings)

1 bag (12-ounce) of cranberries (rinsed and drained)

2-3 jalapeno peppers (seeded and minced)

1 teaspoons of freshly squeezed lemon juice

1/4 cup of dark wine

A cup of water

3/4 cup of sugar

DIRECTIONS (PREP + COOK TIME: 17 MINUTES)

Mix all the ingredients in your Foodi and stir to dissolve the sugar. Close the pressure lid and cook on high mode for 10 minutes. Let the accumulated vapor exit naturally for 10 minutes and quick release the rest. Puree the contents partially and simmer on sauté mode until it thickens. Cool and serve. You can refrigerate the leftovers for two weeks.

Silky Creamy Chicken Mulligatawny Soup

INGREDIENTS (8 Servings)

4 tablespoons of unsalted butter

1 small onion, chopped

1" fresh ginger herb, minced

1 celery stalk, chopped

2 small carrots, diced

2 teaspoons of curry powder

½ teaspoons of black pepper, freshly ground

1 teaspoon of sea salt

1/8 teaspoon of ground nutmeg

1/8 teaspoon of dried thyme

8 chicken thighs (bony but skinless)

3 cups of chicken broth

2 cups of cauliflower florets, minced

2 cups of coconut milk full fat

¼ cup of fresh cilantro chopped, plus more for garnishing

DIRECTIONS (PREP + COOK TIME: 45 MINUTES)

Preheat the unit on sauté mode. Melt the butter and add the onions and garlic. Cook the onions until they soften. Add the carrots and celery and cook while stirring for a minute. Add the remaining ingredients (except cilantro and coconut milk) and close the pressure lid. Cook the mixture on high mode for fifteen minutes. Quick release the in-built steam and open the lid. Add the coconut milk and cilantro. Stir. Serve your soup while garnished with cilantro.

Ethiopian Spinach Lentil Soup

INGREDIENTS (5 Servings)

6 ounces of spinach

2 cups of lentils

8 glasses of water

1 medium red onion, chopped finely

4 tablespoons of lemon juice

1 tablespoon of essential olive oil

2 tablespoons of unsalted butter

2 teaspoons of ground coriander

2 teaspoons of salt

½ teaspoon of turmeric powder

1 teaspoon of garlic powder

½ teaspoon of cinnamon powder

¼ teaspoon of cayenne pepper

¼ teaspoon of pepper

¼ teaspoon of fresh nutmeg, grated

¼ teaspoon of cardamom powder

¼ teaspoon of clove powder

DIRECTIONS (PREP + COOK TIME: 25 MINUTES)

Preheat the unit on sauté mode. Heat the oil and butter. Add all the herbs and spices (except the fresh lemon juice, salt, and pepper) and cook for 3 minutes. Add water and lentils. Stir and close the pressure lid. Cook everything on high mode for 10 minutes. Let the in-built vapor exit naturally for 10 minutes and quick release the rest. Season your lentil soup with salt and pepper. Add spinach and the fresh lemon juice. Stir and serve hot.

Conclusion

Did you delight in attempting these brand-new and also scrumptious recipes?

However we have actually come to the end of this cookbook regarding using the fantastic Ninja Foodi multi-cooker, which I really wish you delighted in.

To improve your wellness we would love to encourage you to combine physical activity and a dynamic way of living along with following these superb recipes, so as to accentuate the renovations. we will certainly be back quickly with a growing number of intriguing vegetarian dishes, a large hug, see you soon.